HEART HEALTH TODAY

IT'S MORE THAN BLOOD PRESSURE AND CHOLESTEROL

6 Simple Ways to Improve Our Heart Health Now

DONALD ZONE, M.D., F.A.C.C.
with the Heart Health Today Team

TO THE AMAZING LINDA —
YOU ARE AN INSPIRATION TO US ALL —
AND FUN TO BOOT —
BEST HEART HEALTH ALWAYS —
DON

ACKNOWLEDGEMENTS

Great credit is due to all those who teach. Family, school teachers, friends, and colleagues all teach us much. We have found that those only one or two steps ahead of us often teach us the most.

In the field of human health, we are privileged to give our perspective on the absolute wealth of information presented by innumerable contributors. We are thankful to them for sharing via the multitude of journals, conferences, media presentations, and conversations we enjoy.

DEDICATION

TO MY PARENTS, whose values are timeless and perseverance inspiring.

TO OUR AMAZING FAMILY, especially ML, who always support and encourage all of us.

TO OUR TEACHERS, who demonstrated the distinct path to understanding.

TO OUR FRIENDS, COLLEAGUES, AND CLASSMATES, who continue to inspire and amaze us.

DISCLAIMER

This book is designed to provide our perspective on useful information. This publication is not meant to be used, nor should it be used, to diagnose or treat any medical condition. That is a matter between you and your own health care provider. Neither the publisher or authors are responsible for any specific health needs, including but not limited to allergies that may require medical attention and likewise are not liable for any damages or negative consequences from any treatment, action, application, or preparation to any person reading or following the information provided herein. References are provided for informational purposes only and do not constitute endorsement of any sources. For a more complete understanding of this, consult the disclaimer at the end of this book.

TABLE OF CONTENTS

INTRODUCTION

Why We Do This

Recently, I had some electrical work that needed to be done. A solid, salt-of-the-earth type of guy arrived. This electrician obviously knew what he was doing and had a lot going for him. He was very personable, made a good living, and seemed like an involved father (he was picking his daughter up from basketball practice later that day). On the other hand, he was overweight, smelled of cigarettes, ate lots of fast food, and even boasted a bit about that lifestyle. I suggested during our banter that he was likely on his way to a bad heart outcome at some point. He just casually joked that I would be the first one he called if he did.

This worker's personal pickup truck was amazing—shiny, neat, and obviously his most prized possession. He took much better care of his pickup than he did of himself! This man had received absolutely no benefit from the recent science on heart health.

~~~

Have you ever noticed that all you learn about your heart health from a standard checkup are your blood pressure and cholesterol levels?

Do you realize that the common knowledge about heart disease is quite often sadly outdated and often just plain incorrect?

Have you or any of your relatives, friends, or acquaintances been affected by heart attack, stroke, or aneurysm?

Have you independently sought out information to help you live a healthier lifestyle because of the pain and suffering you have seen this disease cause?

Are you ready to receive and implement the most current information on actionable items that can start to improve your heart health today?

~~~

Hi! I'm Dr. Don Zone, the founder of Heart Health Today. Overcoming the curse of heart disease has been a lifelong quest of mine. Like many of you, I have seen loved ones suffer or die from the many manifestations of blockage or rupture of arteries. Those manifestations paint a picture of chest pain, shortness of breath, fatigue, swelling, lightheadedness, passing out, and the continuing fear of another heart event.

The probability of having heart or blood vessel disease is huge. We don't need to review all of the extensive data to be convinced that heart disease, stroke, and diabetes ridiculously outrank all forms of cancer combined as the leading cause of disability and death in our society today.

In this book, our Heart Health Today's amazing team addresses 6 determinants of our heart and blood vessels' health. We point to effective, simple measures available to everyone. Plaque buildup in arteries leads to heart attacks, strokes, aneurysms, and limb loss. This is preventable, can be arrested, and is indeed reversible.

One of my earliest memories is accompanying my M.D. father back when doctors actually made house calls. We came into a home with our black bag, heavy with a blood pressure cuff, stethoscope, sterile syringes, cotton balls, antiseptics, vials of penicillin, and other injectables as well as several bottles of pills. We saw very clearly how a person's disease affected their lives. Some lived from bed to bathroom having suffered a stroke. Some needed nitroglycerine for their chest pain. Others could only walk a few feet because of their heart failure. Our weak water shots managed to relieve some of the swelling in their belly and feet but all too often, our treatments were only minimally effective.

At other times, all we had to offer was comfort and consolation. We were there just to confirm the obvious, that a loved one had succumbed to a vicious disease that tragically struck without warning.

My work in medical school and as a board-certified cardiologist allowed me to employ tremendous new treatments for heart disease. Giving ever-improving medicines that held the enemy at bay has been a privilege. The scientific advances that have occurred through the years have been truly fantastic.

I was in awe when I first saw a heart attack victim have his artery unplugged with a wire and balloon by Andreas Gruentzig, the first person to ever do such a thing. As thirty or so of us watched from the gallery, the screen showed the X-Ray image of a thin wire poking through the blockage. Life-sustaining blood began to flow, halting the heart attack in its tracks. The electrifying cheer that erupted from those of us watching was a unique thrill of a lifetime. The procedure was beyond revolutionary. Participating in the progress of the techniques of angioplasty and stents was most gratifying.

As important and lifesaving as that work is, I realized after over forty wonderful years in the field, that I was still a 911 doc, a fireman trying to put out or contain a fire already well underway. I knew that stopping the disease at its root causes and even reversing it is what I would focus on next.

My aha moment came a few years ago when I was attending a conference where some of the top researchers in the world were speaking about the very latest results in prevention and reversal of vascular disease. I happened to sit down for lunch at a round table with five of the top people in the field. One of them was the person who had just presented a fantastic research paper showing reversal of plaques blocking human arteries. Somewhat naively, I commented on how most people don't appreciate that such a thing is even possible. His reply was direct and curt, "We showed that several years ago."

I was quiet as the rest of lunch was filled with these researchers discussing their latest ideas and pending research grants.

As I returned to my hotel room and reflected on this experience, I realized that it is the tremendous biological research that has enabled stupendous progress to occur in our understanding of this disease. I was very bluntly struck, however, that while this current information is readily shared among the researchers and top healthcare professionals, things slow down dramatically as information works its way through the multiple tiers of our health delivery system. What is sadly lacking is a stronger, direct connection between the research information and those who have chosen other paths in life.

House calls still have their place. I know that each home can greatly benefit from knowing what can currently be done to lessen and even avoid the impact of this sneaky villain known as heart disease.

In this book, my team and I enumerate 6 basic actions we can take. All are based on current scientific evidence of their ability to improve cardiovascular health, live life more fully, and avoid the potentially catastrophic suffering associated with this wicked disease.

Today's doctor is often only allotted 12 to 15 minutes for a follow-up patient. At the very least 5 minutes are spent on the computer with the electronic medical record. That leaves less than 10 minutes to listen to the symptoms, do an exam, assess the effect of any therapy, order any appropriate tests, and write any applicable prescriptions. All too often, the basics of prevention are reduced to a quick phrase imparted while walking out the door, "And by the way, make sure you eat a good diet and get exercise."

Diet and exercise—two of the most dreaded words in the English language. We think activity and nutrition are much more motivating names for two of the most important health habits.

What we explain here are 6 areas that clearly should be addressed with everyone, but quite often get less attention than they deserve. Our first reviewers said they didn't realize these simple actions were scientifically shown to be so effective. They felt relieved to know they were taking advantage of the very latest research available.

We promise that using this information can upgrade your heart health to today's standards in just a few short weeks.

~~~

Like the overweight smoker I met with the immaculately well-cared for truck, we all know people who meticulously care for their house, yard, apartment or pet, all the while neglecting themselves. Our attitude toward our optimal health matters. Let's not be the one who puts maintenance of our possessions above maintenance of ourselves.

Likewise, don't be the one who keeps putting this off and then only responds in the crisis situation. Taking action now can avoid much grief in the future. What can be done later, do now. What can be done tomorrow, do today.

There are a huge number of things we can do to improve our heart health. Some measures, which have reached the public media, are of course bogus or minimally effective at best. Some, however, can be truly effective. We report further on applying the real advances most effectively to our lives at hearthealthtoday.com

Here, we have distilled down what we feel are the 6 most important actions we can take as individuals today to address this huge problem and allow us to more fully enjoy the many other areas we wish to pursue in life:

1. Reduce harmful inflammation

2. Change some of the DNA within our bodies—yes, we will confirm that this is true

3. Maintain healthy activity

4. Optimize a critical step in our nutrition

5. Optimize one of the most important hormones in our body

6. Optimize the most beneficial fat in our system

In the following chapters we use an easy-to-follow format:

I CAN DO

I FOR REDUCING HARMFUL INFLAMMATION

C FOR CONTROLLING GUT HEALTH

A FOR ACTIVITY

N FOR GOOD NUTRITION

D FOR OPTIMAL VITAMIN D3 LEVELS

O FOR OPTIMAL OMEGA 3 LEVELS

~~~

As always, the most important thing is to DO, so we will address those first.

WE ALL CAN DO.

We must take control of this risk in our lives, so we can get on with the rest.

Let's achieve our best heart health always,

DZ and HHT team

D3 VITAMIN

GOD RIGHT FROM THE START

And God said, "Let there be light"; and there was light. And God saw that the light was good." (Genesis 1:3-4, ESV).

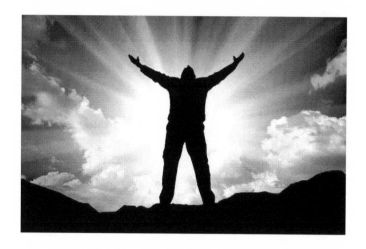

The Higher Power Right from the Start

D3 vitamin at optimal levels is critical for heart health

Our perspective: foods and sunshine might not be the most practical or best sources.

<u>Background</u>

Light, of course, existed before humans. It does not come naturally to think that the health of our heart and its system of arteries is tremendously impacted by sunlight. The link just doesn't immediately spring to mind. However, the connection is that sunlight, specifically the UVB rays, acts on skin cells to produce a substance that is absolutely integral to heart health.

In the 1920s, Elmer McCollum and others were investigating cod liver oil when they isolated this factor. Being the fourth such substance to be identified, it was simply named vitamin D.

Today we know oh so much more!

1. It is actually a hormone, not a vitamin

Hormone—a regulatory substance produced in an organism and transported in tissue fluids such as blood…to stimulate specific cells or tissues into action.

2. Sunshine, the skin, the liver, the intestine, the kidney, and other hormones all play a part in the way we handle vitamin D.

We humans have a great variability in our vitamin D hormone levels since the effectiveness of each of these steps is so very different from person to person. (See Drill Down 1)

3. Vitamin D is critical in our system.

There are over 100,000 biochemical reactions that comprise our human biology. Over 50,000 of these are known to require the presence of vitamin D. Activated vitamin D is absolutely essential for the optimal functioning of these multiple biochemical reactions occurring each second in every cell of our bodies.

4. The level of vitamin D in our system matters.

Multiple scientific investigations have shown that there are bad, good, very good, and optimal levels of vitamin D

5. Low vitamin D levels are unfortunately very common in our society.

A predominantly *indoor lifestyle* or just *living in the north* almost ensures we will have an inadequate level of vitamin D. This is especially true during the *winter* months. Likewise, if our diet resembles the standard American diet (S.A.D.), we are also very likely to have a low vitamin D level.

6. Vitamin D can be easily measured in the blood.

Heart Health Importance of Vitamin D

Consider the following:

Deficient levels of vitamin D roughly double the risk of heart attack in previously healthy individuals. (2)

Low vitamin D levels are associated with high blood pressure (5)

The risk of preeclampsia (dangerously high blood pressure in pregnancy) is doubled in those with low vitamin D levels. (4)

Supplementation with vitamin D has been shown to improve high blood pressure (hypertension.) (9)

We see that maintaining optimal levels of vitamin D is clearly a key to optimal heart health.

The Problem with Sunlight as a Source of Vitamin D

The skin makes vitamin D when it is exposed to UVB rays of sunlight, making vitamin D popularly known as the "sunshine vitamin." However, UVB rays in sunlight cause skin cancers.

So there is a huge problem with using sunlight as a major source of vitamin D. These UVB rays can damage the DNA in skin cells, causing various forms of skin cancer. Most notable of these is the deadly type, melanoma.

Dermatologists commonly recommend severely limiting sunlight exposure for this reason.

Using high SPF sunscreens has become a standard in our society. All the while, however, too little sunlight and too little vitamin D are ruining our heart health.

The Multiple Actions of Vitamin D

We think it's worth digressing from the heart health theme for a minute to consider that it's not only the heart and blood vessels that are impacted by less than optimal levels of vitamin D. An optimal vitamin D level is needed for an optimally functioning human.

It is so important to health that some have advocated changing the old terminology and referring to it more correctly as a hormone, prohormone or even a "vitamone."

The most well-known action of this hormone is to build bones. There are, however, multiple other actions of this critical substance, which has a crucial role throughout our bodies. When we have low levels of vitamin D, our body objects, responds poorly, and we begin to recognize more and more of the various symptoms.

For example, fatigue, osteoporosis, poor eyesight, and an absolute myriad of other symptoms and disorders can be caused by low vitamin D levels. (2, 3) Notably, many mental problems including depression, seasonal affective disorder, sleep disturbances, "brain fog," and mood disturbances are associated with low vitamin D levels. For example, pediatricians have an insightful characterization of sick babies and children that simply appear ill from unclear causes. They call it "failure to thrive." Failure to thrive, or just feeling punk, is one of the ways a less-than-optimal vitamin D level manifests itself.

We must allow the many biochemical reactions requiring vitamin D to function at their very best! Let's clear some of those symptoms by maintaining an optimal vitamin D level.

The Human Spirit

Although we may tend to think of the mind and body separately, we must realize that biologically they are similarly functioning huge sets of biochemical reactions, requiring the right balance of nutrients to function at their best. That said, this biological reality should not be confused with the human spirit. Our spirituality is beyond the scope of this book.

Food as a Source of Vitamin D

Food is a good source of vitamin D, but while searching for an optimal amount of vitamin D in food is possible, it can be difficult to do this safely or practically. We will often have to accept many ugly ingredients or unfamiliar foods in the process.

One of the best food sources of vitamin D is fatty fish, including halibut, salmon, tuna, trout, and catfish. Other good sources, although uncommon in American diets, include herring, sardines, and mackerel.

Sources of vitamin D include:

- halibut

- salmon

- tuna

- trout

- catfish

- mackerel

- herring

- sardines

- shiitake and button mushrooms

When choosing fish, we must be careful that they come from uncontaminated waters to avoid taking in mercury and other toxins along with the fish. Mercury accumulates in fish living in the contaminated waters of the coasts and the Great Lakes.

It's worth repeating that mercury is an absolute toxin! (1) It has no useful role in human biology. Mercury's poisonous effects are manifested most clearly in neurological and behavioral abnormalities. Likewise, the heart and arteries are not immune from mercury's toxic effects. This element's ability to cause high blood pressure and damage to the delicate inner lining of blood vessels has been clearly proven.(6)

On a positive note, one common and relatively safe source of vitamin D is mushrooms. Shiitake and button mushrooms are naturally high in vitamin D.

Obviously, the overall problem here is that in order to get optimal vitamin D from food alone, we may have to accept many ugly ingredients and unfamiliar foods in the process.

Foods Supplemented with Vitamin D

Fortified foods and multiple vitamins are OK but typically contain only small amounts of vitamin D.

Several decades ago, the U.S. Government began recommending that cow milk be supplemented with vitamin D. Poor bone growth (rickets) had been identified in children deficient in this factor. The common, major manifestations of the disorder were improved by this "fortification." Other products such as almond milk, soy milk, and tofu have followed suit.

Unfortunately, many commonly advertised food sources have so little vitamin D that they only allow us to maintain subsistence levels. Considering a daily vitamin D intake of 5,000 to 10,000 IU from all sources, we get only:

100 IU from 1 cup of fortified milk
40 IU from on large egg
130 IU from 1 oz. of canned salmon
65 IU from 1 oz. of light canned tuna
80 IU from 6 oz. of fortified yogurt
40 IU from one cup of fortified cereal

440 IU from 3 oz. of sockeye salmon
600 TO 1,000 IU in a typical multivitamin

Other branded food sources that have added vitamin D to their formulations include many branded cereal products, yogurts, and juices. However, many of these products that provide some good (vitamin D, calcium) also pack in the nutritionally ugly (loads of sugar, high fructose corn syrup, artificial sweeteners etc.).

We Are All Unique. One Dose Does Not Fit All.

As if all these factors don't make the situation complicated enough, the optimal amount to take varies tremendously from person to person. Many variables determine vitamin D blood levels including an individual's skin color as well as their recent amount of sunlight exposure.

Additionally, the liver must convert D3 to a circulating form, and liver function varies from person to person. The kidney converts the circulating form to the active form and individual kidney function is variable.

Other variables related to oral intake of vitamin D include diet, gut absorption capabilities, and the amount of fat intake. (Vitamin D is fat soluble and gets absorbed with the fats in food.)

All these problems have caused many individuals to choose to take vitamin D as a capsule or spray as part of their daily regimen.

What Form of Vitamin D Do We Want?

The skin makes the D3 form of vitamin D. This is the more potent form and preferred for that reason. Food sources and supplements may include the D2 as well as the D3 form. Providers of vitamin D have predominantly chosen D3 at this point.

How Much Vitamin D Should We Get?

Some sources quote guesstimates for a suggested daily oral intake for the average person. Commonly, these suggested amounts are based on very old information regarding the amount needed to prevent rickets in children. Those levels are not the best ones to prevent heart disease. Recommendations designed to avoid clear deficiency are different than those designed to achieve an optimal level.

The recommended daily allowances quoted on processed food products (600 to 800 IU per day) are unlikely to result in vitamin D levels recommended by most current research on heart disease prevention. A major problem here is that these recommendations are for the "general population," or the theoretical average person. Again, it is abundantly clear that we are all unique with such tremendous person-to-person variability in this regard that these types of recommendations frequently fall short.

In the average adult who does not choose to measure D3 in the blood, we have seen recent recommendation of a 2000 IU supplement or 5000-8000 IU per day from all sources including sunlight, food, and supplements.

Action

We strive to maintain an optimal level of vitamin D in our blood by limiting sunlight exposure to low levels while getting optimal amounts of vitamin D from natural and uncontaminated food sources. While perhaps preferable, this way can, of course, be challenging and fall short in letting us achieve our optimal blood level. The less sunlight we receive, the more we must get from food and supplemental sources.

As we discussed, Vitamin D can be supplemented orally with capsules, tablets, or sprays. This method avoids the problem inherent in sunlight and food sources.

Blood test measurements facilitate maintaining an effective and safe range. Presently, authorities suggest that optimal levels are in the range of 60 to 80 ng/ml. Levels below 30 are clearly deficient.

We must definitely get our vitamin D level measured. We must all strive to be sure our health care provider includes vitamin D in our blood tests. Annual measurements are good, and seasonal measurements at the end of winter and summer are even more helpful.

This may be best measured as vitamin D 25 OH total (D2+D3).

LESS THAN 30=DEFICIENT
30 TO 40 = JUST ADEQUATE
40 TO 60= BETTER
60 TO 80= OPTIMAL

Supplementation up to 5000 IU per day may well be necessary to attain optimal levels. Those with autoimmune disease may require even more.

Your healthcare professional will be able to help us with this. If for any reason that does not work well, home testing kits are a readily available and accurate way to manage our own vitamin D level. Remember that the right dose of vitamin D is the one that maintains the optimal blood level.

There is some rationale for getting a portion of our vitamin D from sunlight. Many of us do because of where and how we live. We do of course run a risk of skin cancer whenever we do so. Some experts recommend 15-30 minutes per day between 10:00 and

3:00 p.m. over face, arms, legs or back. To clarify this, more research is needed in determining the role of vitamin D receptors in disease processes.

Caution: We do not take supplements of over 5000 IU per day without a specific recommendation from our doctor. It is very unlikely, but perhaps possible, to take too much vitamin D, so we check blood levels and not overdo the dose.

The vitamin D council has very good guidelines and visiting this link is a very reasonable choice. (See Drill Down 2)

~~~

Is achieving an optimal level of vitamin D important enough to warrant this amount of effort? Absolutely it is. We suggest that based on today's knowledge, maintaining an optimal vitamin D3 level of 60 to 80 ng/ml is critical to our heart health. Our perspective is that supplementation with vitamin D3 is the most practical way to improve this crucial aspect of our heart health.

Most of us know that omega-3 foods are good for our heart and blood vessels, but do we need to buy brightly labeled packaged foods to get some? Clearly there are simpler ways. We review that next.

~~~

DRILL DOWNS

Drill Down 1:

Vitamin D3 (cholecalciferol) is made by the skin as it interacts with sunshine. It also occurs naturally in some foods. It is then modified in the liver to the circulating form (25 hydroxy cholecalciferol) and with the help of parathyroid hormone is converted in the kidney to the activated form (1,25 dihydroxycholecalciferol).

Drill Down 2:

http://vitamind3-cholecalciferol.com/vitamin-d-dosage

http://www.vitamindcouncil.org/

~~~

Most of us know omega-3s are good for us. In addition to the brightly labeled package foods, there are many simple ways to improve our omega-3 intake.

Next, we'll take a look at these possibilities. A reasonable way to measure our results is also available.

~~~

References and Further Reading:

1. Arch Intern Med. 2009; 169(6): 626-632

2. Wang TJ, Pencina MJ, Booth SL, et al. Vitamin D deficiency and risk of cardiovascular disease. Circulation. 2008;117:503–11. [PMC free article] [PubMed]

3. Pilz S, März W, Wellnitz B, et al. Association of vitamin D deficiency with heart failure and sudden cardiac death in a large cross-sectional study of patients referred for coronary angiography. J Clin Endocrinol Metab. 2008;93:3927–35 [PubMed]

4. Sasan, S.B. et al. Clinical Study The Effects of Vitamin D Supplement on Prevention of Recurrence of Preeclampsia in Pregnant Women with a History of Preeclampsia. Obstetrics and Gynecology International, 2017

5. Forman JP, Giovannucci E, Holmes MD, et al. Plasma 25-hydroxyvitamin D levels and risk of incident hypertension. Hypertension. 2007;49:1063–9 [PubMed]

6. Aggarwal, Nisha & P. Reis, Jared & Michos, Erin. (2010). Vitamin D Deficiency and Its Implications on Cardiovascular Disease. Current Cardiovascular Risk Reports.2010; 4(1):68-75. 10.1007/s12170-009-0072-1

7. Vitamin D Fact Sheet for Health Professionals, ods.od.nih.gov

8. Kunutsor, S. K. et al. Vitamin D and risk of future hypertension: meta-analysis of 283,537 participants. European Journal of Epidemiology 2013;28;205-221

9. Carrara, D. et al. Cholecalciferol administration blunts the systemic renin angiotensin system in essential hypertensives with hypovitaminosis D. Journal of the renin angiotensin aldosterone system 2013;15;82-87

OMEGA-3S

A NEW KEY TO HEART HEALTH

Then God said, "Let the oceans swarm with living creatures." (Genesis 1:20, International Standard Version).

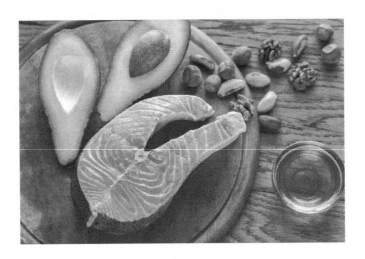

Consider Maintaining an Optimal Omega-3 Index (8% or greater)

In the past few years, some studies have shown omega-3s are associated with decreased heart disease and optimal heart health. Maintaining an optimal intake of this building block of the heart and blood vessels can be a key part of a heart-healthy life.

Studies have linked omega-3s to lower risk of artery blockage (plaque), fewer abnormal heartbeats (arrhythmias), lower blood pressure, and lower bad fats in the blood.

A study from Jan 2017 looked at data regarding omega-3 and heart disease. (2) Looking back at studies of populations, the authors found that two omega-3 fatty acids (EPA & DHA) were clearly beneficial in those with elevated triglycerides and elevated LDL cholesterol. The improvement was 16% in those with triglycerides over 150 and a 14% improvement in those with LDL above 130.

We are aware of large collections of self-reported diet and variable dose studies which fail to show a benefit, but continue to conclude that properly dosed and measured in the individual, omega-3s are heart healthy.

Of course, it all started with light (Genesis1: 3-4) and the subsequent appearance of simple plants we call algae. Algae, as we know, use the sunlight and carbon dioxide in the air and produce water and oxygen via the process of photosynthesis. Algae then progressed to produce complex molecules, among them a type we know as omega-3s.

Some species at various points in the food chain have concentrated this nutrient extremely well. Micro marine life depends on algae as a food source and krill (a mini shrimp) is known to concentrate omega-3s especially well. Some large fish at the top of the food chain also concentrate significant amounts of omega-3s.

One of the richest human food sources of this critical nutrient is cold water fish. Salmon, bluefin tuna, cod, and some other large fish are generally good sources of omega-3s, depending somewhat on where they live and eat.

Cows, chickens, and other animals concentrate omega-3 to a lesser degree, also depending on their food source. Chickens fed omega-3 rich feed produce eggs with a high content of this nutrient. Likewise, grass-fed beef is also higher in omega-3 than grain fed. By now, most of us have seen these and other highly advertised products in our restaurants and grocery stores.

How do we know we are taking maximum advantage of this scientific breakthrough? One way presently available is to maintain an optimal omega-3 index.

Maintain an Optimal Omega-3 Index.

This is our perspective on one thing we can do as individuals that may well improve our heart health. Omega-3 is the last in the I CAN DO acronym, but nonetheless quite important. The index is not a perfect measure for sure, but from our view is one of the best we have available to us today.

Remember that omega-3s is a category of fats, but more importantly are **GOOD FATS.**

Optimal levels of the right omega-3s, EPA and DHA, in our system result in amazingly well-functioning blood vessels and heart. (See Drill Down 1)

We endeavor to increase Omega-3s in the diet, decreasing Omega-6 and avoiding trans fat altogether.

How We Get Omega-3S

With some fats, such as omega-3 and trans fats, our blood levels are increased directly by the amount we eat. Importantly, we must understand that this is distinctly different from saturated fat which is raised by excess sugars and non-vegetable carbohydrate. It's just the way our biochemistry works.

As most of us clearly know, our nutrition has deteriorated over the past several decades. Loads of sugar and nutrient-sparse foods abound. An optimal ratio of omega-6 to omega-3 in our nutrition is estimated at 4 to 1 or less. Quite unfortunately, our present-day STANDARD AMERICAN DIET (S.A.D.) CONTAINS A RATIO OF 25 to 1.

The other stubborn fact is that there are fatty acids we need but cannot make by ourselves, these are so-called "essential fatty acids." They are ALA and Linoleic acid, which are available from vegetable sources and must be consumed in the diet. However, there is another stubborn fact. THE HUMAN LIVER CAN ONLY CONVERT A SMALL PERCENTAGE OF THESE TO THE DESIRED EPA AND DHA. It is thus best to consume EPA and DHA directly. This can take many forms including fish, fish oil, krill oil or direct algal sources.

The recent good news, especially for those choosing a vegan diet, is that algal EPA & DHA derived from algae is now available in capsules and provide an excellent source of these omega-3s. This is of course not only for vegans. Any one of us can get our DHA and EPA this way if we wish and not have to rely on fish or seafood based sources. (See Drill Down 2)

Biochemistry Is the Key

Refer to Drill Down 3 for details on the ARA or arachidonic acid pathway. Generally speaking, omega-6s need to be kept under control.

The omega-3 construction sequence meanwhile produces the opposite, anti-inflammatory molecules, cutting down on unnecessary and heart-damaging inflammation.

Trans Fat

So if omega-3s are the beneficial fats, which are the bad ones?

Omega-6 biology produces inflammatory molecules.

A good level of these is necessary to repair injured areas of the body. Omega-6-produced molecules rush to injured sites to initiate the healing process or fend off harmful bacteria. This is all well and good.

One grossly simplified visual that can allow us to remember that trans fats are bad is to think of them as having sharp edges like tire spikes, biting into and damaging the road.

The opposite of trans is "cis."

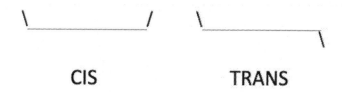

Trans fats do not occur naturally and should be avoided. Do not eat processed foods. Eat whole, fresh food. (2)

To understand how clear this recommendation is, we should appreciate that the U.S. Government has acted to remove trans fat from the food supply by 2018.

It's so good to see a government working in a good way!

Lipids and Heart Disease

Let's be clear that the lipid role in cardiovascular disease is very important. What we must do, however, is make sure it is understood with today's knowledge.

Long-chain polyunsaturated omega-3 fatty acids EPA and DHA which come from marine sources are the key. The shorter chain ALA found in plant sources plays a less important role.

Enough EPA/DHA to add is likely about 1 to 1.5 grams. (1,000 to 1,500 milligrams). Supplements up to 3 grams per day have been studied with no significant bad effects being noted. Consult labels and remember that it takes more grams of fish oil to provide the desired grams of EPA/DHA. Also, pay attention to the "serving size" i.e. How many capsules are needed to provide the grams of EPA/DHA listed.

Those who choose krill as a source of omega-3s should note that it is likely the largest animal biomass in the world and thus quite unlikely to be significantly depleted by harvesting it as a food source. The largest plant biomass is phytoplankton, just below krill in the food chain. Krill also provides astaxanthin, a potent antioxidant.

We now know that there are types of fats (omega-3, some 6,7, and 9) that are very good for human nutrition. Our heart health follows.

SOME SOURCES OF OMEGA-3 FATS ARE:

- SALMON
- CRAB
- SHRIMP
- COD
- TILAPIA
- BLUEFIN TUNA
- SCALLOPS
- KRILL OIL
- OMEGA-3 EGGS
- WALNUTS
- ALMOND MILK
- CRUCIFEROUS VEGETABLES—CAULIFLOWER, BROCCOLI
- SPINACH
- ARUGULA
- BEANS
- FOODS FORTIFIED WITH OMEGA-3 FROM ALGAE
- EXTRA VIRGIN OLIVE OIL—If we choose a program including oils, consider keeping extra virgin olive oil handy and put in on whatever seems good to you. Consider olive oil as the primary oil in your kitchen. Shop around, as they have many different tastes. Pick the one you like best. Some specialty stores will let you taste test various products.

Eat omega-3 and similar type fats. Find ways to enjoy and thrive with good nutrition.

CAUTION. We should note that krill is a shellfish and should not be used by those of us who may be allergic to shellfish. Fish and fish oils should be avoided or used with caution in those taking a blood thinning medication. We must check with our health care professional. We should, of course, follow ALL precautions on ANY product label.

We have found a useful link to sensible fish consumption:
www.fda.gov/downloads/Food/ResourcesForYou/

The Power of Positive Thinking

It's best to be positive. Just seek out and eat good foods, and don't spend energy worrying or dwelling on what the bad foods are.

~~~

DRILL DOWNS

Drill Down 1:

Of course, it's the whole human, body, and mind, that functions well given the optimal levels of these molecules. Less than optimal levels of omega-3s result in a more poorly functioning heart, body, and mind. It's progressive, so that when levels are very inadequate, symptoms are more severe.

Drill Down 2:

We can drill down on the biochemistry if we want:

Omega-3s are organic molecules with a double bond on the third carbon from the end of the chain. Thus the term omega (the last letter of the Greek alphabet) and 3 (third from the end).

Let's review some technical information in our drill down:
"Omega-3 Fatty Acids and Health: Fact Sheet for Health Professionals". US National Institutes of Health, Office of Dietary Supplements. 2 November 2016.

> *"The human body can only form carbon–carbon double bonds after the 9th carbon from the methyl end of a fatty acid [1]. Therefore, ALA and linoleic acid are considered essential fatty acids, meaning that they must be obtained from the diet [2]. ALA can be converted into EPA and then to DHA, but the conversion (which occurs primarily in the liver) is very limited, with reported rates of less than 15% [3]. Therefore, consuming EPA and DHA directly from foods and/or dietary supplements is the only practical way to increase levels of these fatty acids in the body.*

> *ALA is present in plant oils, such as flaxseed, soybean, and canola oils [3]. DHA and EPA are present in fish, fish oils, and krill oils, but they are originally synthesized by microalgae, not by the fish. When fish consume phytoplankton that consumed microalgae, they accumulate the omega-3s in their tissues [3].*

Drill Down 3:

Wikipedia explains some of this complex biochemistry:

"Dietary arachidonic acid and inflammation:

Increased consumption of arachidonic acid will not cause inflammation during normal metabolic conditions unless lipid peroxidation products are mixed in. Arachidonic acid is metabolized to both proinflammatory and anti-inflammatory eicosanoids during and after the inflammatory response, respectively. Arachidonic acid is also metabolized to inflammatory and anti-inflammatory eicosanoids during and after physical activity to promote growth. However chronic inflammation from exogenous toxins and excessive exercise should not be confused with acute inflammation from exercise and sufficient rest that is required by the inflammatory response to promote the repair and growth of the micro tears of tissues.[32]

However, the evidence is mixed. Some studies giving between 840 mg and 2,000 mg per day to healthy individuals for up to 50 days have shown no increases in inflammation or related metabolic activities.[32][33][34][35] However, others show that increased arachidonic acid levels are actually associated with reduced proinflammatory IL-6 and IL-1 levels and increased anti-inflammatory tumor necrosis factor-beta.[36] This may result in a reduction in systemic inflammation.[medical citation needed]

Arachidonic acid does still play a central role in inflammation related to injury and many diseased states. How it is metabolized in the body dictates its inflammatory or anti-inflammatory activity. Individuals suffering from joint pains or active inflammatory disease may find that increased arachidonic acid consumption exacerbates symptoms, presumably because it is being more readily converted to inflammatory compounds[medical citation needed]. Likewise, high arachidonic acid consumption is not advised for individuals with a history of inflammatory disease, or who are in compromised health. Of note, while ARA supplementation does not appear to have proinflammatory effects in healthy individuals, it may counter the anti-inflammatory effects of omega-3 fatty acid supplementation."[37]

~~~

Do we have biological fires burning out of control within us, destroying our heart health? If so, can we control them? We address this next. Clue: the answer to both questions is "yes."

~~~

References and Suggested Reading:

1. http://www.livescience.com/3505-chemistry-life-human-body.html actually approximately 96% of body mass is carbon, hydrogen, oxygen and nitrogen

2. A Meta-Analysis of Randomized Controlled Trials and Prospective Cohort Studies of Eicosapentaenoic and Docosahexaenoic Long-Chain Omega-3 Fatty Acids and Coronary Heart Disease Risk Alexander, Dominik D. et al. Mayo Clinic Proceedings, Volume 92 , Issue 1, 15–29

3. Has, Petter-Arnt & Wang, Xiaoli & Xiao, Yong-Fu. (2017). Effects of a purified krill oil phospholipid-rich in long-chain omega-3 fatty acids on cardiovascular disease risk factors in non-human primates with naturally occurring diabetes type-2 and dyslipidemia. Lipids in Health and Disease. 16. 10.1186/s12944-017-0411-z

4. Mozaffarian D, Katan MB, Ascherio A, Stampfer MJ, Willett WC (2006). "Trans Fatty Acids and Cardiovascular Disease". New England Journal of Medicine. 354 (15): 1601–1613. doi:10.1056/NEJMra054035

5. https://www.nih.gov/news-events/news-releases/omega-3-fatty-acids-protect-eyes-against-retinopathy-study-finds

6. JAMAInternMed.2016Aug1;176(8):1155-66.doi:10.1001/jamainternmed.2016.2925

7. Chowdhury, R; Warnakula, S; Kunutsor, S; Crowe, F; Ward, HA; Johnson, L; Franco, OH; Butterworth, AS; Forouhi, NG; Thompson, SG; Khaw, KT; Mozaffarian, D; Danesh, J; Di Angelantonio, E (Mar 18, 2014). "Association of dietary, circulating, and supplement fatty acids with coronary risk: a systematic review and meta-analysis". Annals of Internal Medicine. 160 (6): 398–406. doi:10.7326/M13-1788

9. Omega-3 Index for Heart Health Prof. Dr. C. von Schacky, FAHA, FESC Preventive Cardiology Medizinische Klinik und Poliklinik I Ludwig Maximilians-Universität München Clemens.vonSchacky@med.uni-muenchen.de and Omegametrix, Martinsried C.Vonschacky@omegametrix.eu Newcastle, 07 November 2013

10. JAMA Ophthalmology. 2015 Oct; 133(10): 1171-9

11. https://www.ncbi.nlm.nih.gov/pmc/articles/PMC3593234/pdf/nihms433389.pdf

12. link for mercury content of fish.
UCM536321.pdfhttps://www.fda.gov/downloads/Food/FoodborneIllnessContaminants/Metals/

Suggestions:

Omegaquant.com Sioux Falls, South Dakota has a home finger-prick test for the omega-3 index. Attain 8% or greater.

Look carefully for pure, non-rancid, non-farmed raised, non-mercury-contaminated fish oil. Krill oil is an excellent choice.

INFLAMMATION

PUT OUT THE FIRE

CUT UNNEEDED INFLAMMATION

Several decades ago, medical students were shown these three pictures and asked what disease they had in common.

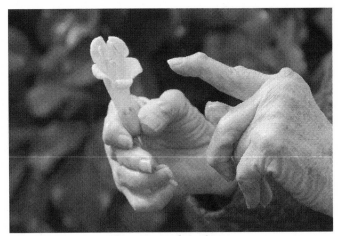

Rheumatoid Arthritis

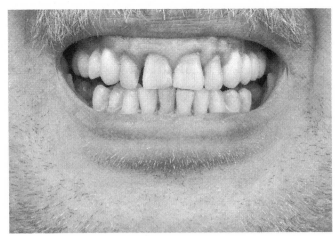

Gingivitis

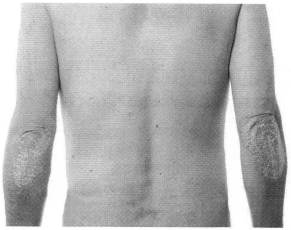

Psoriasis

The unexpected answer is: **HEART DISEASE.**

All three are inflammatory conditions and are associated with an increase in blood vessel damage.

Inflammation is our body's response to harmful events such as physical injury or infections. We all know what happens when we fall and scrape a knee. The involved area becomes red, hot, and tender and may lose some function. A similar inflammatory response occurs with many substances which we inhale, ingest, or contact with our skin or mucous membranes. Think of how our eyes react if we are allergic to pollen.

While the outward manifestation of inflammation may be obvious, the internal consequences aren't intuitively obvious. The unfortunate fact is that inflammation anywhere in our bodies leads to clogged arteries.

Think of the damage that might occur somewhere from fires, windstorms, or floods. First, demolition crews and heavy equipment come in to clean up. As repair and construction proceed, more equipment and construction crews arrive. In the process, the access roads get damaged. Somewhere along those damaged roads, an event may occur that shuts a road down entirely. The roads need to be maintained and repaired.

Our arteries are like roads. They are our transportation system. Our bodies send demolition and construction equipment and crews to sites of damage. In the process, our arteries are slowly damaged. The cracks and potholes in the delicate lining of our blood vessels let in damaging material.

Plaque is an accumulation of destructive material in the wall of the artery. Gradual buildup of plaque results in partial blockage, reduced blood flow, and impaired function of the heart or whichever organ that artery supplies. Bursting of the plaque results in further blockage of the artery. Complete or almost complete blockage produces major bad events.

This is a process that builds up over decades and may start very early in life. Studies from as long ago as the Korean war show this without a doubt.

This process is also well known to occur in all of our blood vessels, not just in one region of the body. Check out anything from the life work of William C. Roberts, MD. He showed conclusively that plaques occur throughout our blood vessels. They are just worse and cause more problems at particular spots like our heart (coronary) arteries.

One medical community calls this problem "plaque disease." That term best states the root cause of most heart and blood vessel disease. Medical professionals use a huge number of names to tell our patients what they have. Most just designate the organ most involved when in actuality all organs are involved. For example, coronary artery disease (CAD) for the heart, peripheral artery disease (PAD) for legs, and carotid artery disease for the neck arteries all refer to the same process of plaque buildup or what is commonly called blockage.

In truth we have a problem with the lining of the miles and miles of blood vessels. Think of how much total road surface there is in your state. Thinking of our bodies like the total road surface in our state will give us a concept of how much blood vessel lining we have. The problem has to be addressed as a whole.

The medical evidence is clear. More inflammation means more plaque.

The firestorm of inflammatory substances scorching the delicate linings of our blood vessels starts the heart attack process.

The Amazingly Good News Is:

1. Inflammation can be controlled.

2. Plaque is reversible.

How Can We Know Our Inflammation Level?

We want inflammation to occur when it is needed to heal an injury or fight off infection. Otherwise, we want very low levels.

Inflammation is well measured by a blood test called hsCRP.

We should regulate our personal program to keep this level low unless inflammation is needed to respond to injury or infection.

Less than 1.0 is good
Less than 0.5 is very good
Less than 0.1 is best

We should monitor our hsCRP level and keep it below 1.0. Find a healthcare professional who will do this with you.

1. Maintain healthy gums. Gum (periodontal) disease is a leading cause of chronic inflammation and is directly related to increased heart disease. Fortunately, and this is very important, newly available electric toothbrushes can do a much better job than our standard brushing habits. (11,12)

2. Maintain a healthy gut. Improve our digestive system with healthy gut bacteria. Probiotics are helpful. Ingest healing substances such as omega-3s to restore the delicate gut lining and decrease the damaged gut that allows too much access for harmful substances into our system.

3. Stop eating substances which cause inflammation. Trans fats in foods, and many ingredients in processed foods, do this. Real, whole foods work best in keeping us healthy. Again, we note that cholesterol and saturated fats are not exactly the enemy here. A plant-based diet may be the best if you choose that challenging path. Consider using only non-inflammatory vegetable oil such as extra virgin olive oil. The substances causing inflammation are somewhat different from person to person. Some people are highly reactive to certain foods or airborne allergens while others are not. Consider pollens, dairy, shellfish, gluten, and many others in this category.

4. Avoid sugary foods because they are inflammatory. Doing this may make us feel uncomfortable, achy, or flu-like for a couple of days only. We can minimize this temporary effect by eating good fatty foods like walnuts, dark chocolate, almonds, macadamia nuts, avocado, guacamole, olive oil, salmon, sea bass, and snapper. You may even eat herring or sardines if you like them. Drinking plenty of water also helps.

5. Eat certain foods, including food concentrates, which naturally decrease inflammation. Among these are nuts, seeds, ginger, garlic, cayenne, extra virgin olive oil, colorful vegetables, and omega-3 sources such as salmon, fish oil and krill.

6. Use curcumin. Curcumin is a component of the spice turmeric. The curcumin component is the most active and studied. Curcumin can significantly reduce the inflammation in our bodies. (13)

7. Keep glutathione levels high. Glutathione is our master antioxidant, recycling antioxidants in our bodies. (14) Keep levels up with the fantastic broccoli family of vegetables, onions, and garlic. Bioactive whey protein helps but must be made from non-denatured protein, non-pasteurized and not from industrially produced milk. Multiple cofactors and nutrients must be supplied in proper amounts to optimize glutathione function.

8. Drink green tea. Drinking green tea can help improve cardiovascular health. The Matcha and Tulsi varieties contain substances which can be especially beneficial.

Bonus Time

Don't be surprised if joint aches and pains and many other symptoms get better. The same mechanism that inflames our blood vessels is involved with all the other systems of our body.

The Devil Is in the Details

And, ahh, yes—the details—like finding fault with one particular food or substance. That is where the devil is. We should not get "off in the weeds" and avoid the clear and obvious path.

Becoming distracted or leaving the path because we see a small stone in our way is always a bad idea. The perfect path, without some bends and twists and minor obstructions, is not known. However, the general direction and choices along the way are abundantly clear. Let's just make them!

We Can Put out the Fire of Heart Disease

Much of the recent elucidation of the role of inflammation in causing heart disease should be credited to the work of Dr. Paul Ridker. He is Director of the Center for Cardiovascular Disease Prevention at Brigham and Women's Hospital in Boston. Delving into his findings are well worthwhile. The reference links we have listed are very enlightening.

~~~

What other major cause of heart disease is not intuitively obvious?

Is our heart health all predetermined in our genes? Or is it possible to change some of our DNA to blunt this cause of heart disease? The answer is: Yes. We know it is.

~~~

References and Further Reading:

1. http://www.Epi.Umn.Edu/cvdepi/study-synopsis/korean-soldiers-study/

2. Ridker pm, et al "antiinflammatory therapy with canakinumab for atherosclerotic disease (cantos)" n engl j med 2017; doi: 10.1056/Nejmoa1707914

3. Francis, Andrew a; Pierce, Grant n (2011). "An integrated approach for the mechanisms responsible for atherosclerotic plaque regression". Experimental & ClinicalCardiology. 16(3):Fall2011:77–86. Issn 1205-6626. Pmc 3209544 . Pmid 22065938

4. Ridker,pm Circulation. 2003;107:363-369
https://doi.Org/10.1161/01.Cir.0000053730.47739.3

5. Kaivan vaidya, Clare Arnott, Gonzalo j. Martínez, Bernard ng, Samuel McCormack, David R. Sullivan, David S. Celermajer, Sanjay Patel
Colchicine therapy and plaque stabilization in patients with acute coronary syndrome. Jacc: cardiovascular imaging, available online 18 october 2017

6. Ridker, PM and Narula, JACC: cardiovascular imaging
October 2017 doi: 10.1016/J.Jcmg.2017.10.001

7. www.NCBI.NLM.NIH.Gov/pubmed/20657536

8. Ridker PM, Rifai N, Pfeffer MA, et al. Inflammation, pravastatin, and the risk of coronary events after myocardial infarction in patients with average cholesterol levels. Cholesterol and recurrent events (care) investigators. Circulation. 1998;98(9):839-844

9. Ridker P. How common is residual inflammatory risk? Circ res. 2017;120:617-619.

10. Huang w. And Glass C. Nuclear receptors and inflammation control: molecular mechanisms and pathophysiological relevance. Arterioscler Thromb vasc biol. 2010; 30(8): 1542–1549

11. Rosma, NA, et. Al. J. Periodontol. 2008 Aug; 79 (8): 1386-94.
Doi: 10.1902/Jop.2008.070654.: Comparison of the use of different modes of Mechanical oral hygiene in prevention of plaque and gingivitis.

12. Nathoo, S, Et. Al.: Comparison of plaque removal efficacy of a battery-powered toothbrush And a manual toothbrush j. Clin. Dent. 2003; 14(2): 34-7

13. Curcumin downregulates human tumor necrosis factor-α levels: a systematic review and meta-analysis of randomized controlled trials.
Sahebkar A, Cicero AFG, Simental-mendía LE, Aggarwal BB, Gupta SC.
Pharmacol res. 2016 May;107:234-242. Doi: 10.1016/J.Phrs.2016.03.026. Epub 2016 mar 26. Review. Pmid: 27025786

14. Bea,F.,Hudson,f.N.,Chait,A. Et al. (2003) Induction of glutathione synthesis in macrophages by oxidized low-density lipoproteins is mediated by consensus antioxidant response elements. Circ.Res,92,386-393

15. https://www.NCBI.NLM.NIH.Gov/pmc/articles/pmc4945585/pdf/wjcc-4-155.Pdf

Control Gut Health

CHANGE OUR DNA

MAINTAIN HEALTHY GUT ORGANISMS

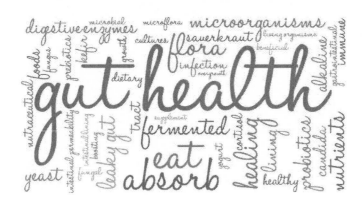

If our nutrient intake system functions poorly at any step, this leads to plaque and heart disease.

Very few, if any, of us would have thought that the particular organisms in our gut are a cause of heart disease, but in fact, they are. Delivering the best nutrients into our cells leads to optimal heart health.

Healthy microorganisms in our gut allow the lining of the gut to carry out its proper function as gatekeeper. It is designed to allow only certain types and sizes of materials into our system. In fact, most of our immune cells are located near the gut lining. Like an army of soldiers, they stand ready to assess what they encounter and eliminate the undesirable types.

Bad microorganisms can lead to a damaged lining of the intestines and poor handling of nutrients. They cause inflammation in our gut, which fuels plaque in our blood vessels.

As we chew food, we break it up and add enzymes to start digestion. The stomach adds other components. Most nutrients are absorbed in the intestines. A critical piece of this breakdown of the raw materials we use to make and maintain ourselves is our own good microorganisms. Yes, our very own bacteria and fungi. Amazing as it is, the number of these in our bodies are equal to or greater than our human cells.

In fact, our bodies contain much more gut bacterial DNA than human DNA. (See Drill Down 1)

In every single cell of our bodies, there are tens of thousands of chemical reactions going on in order to maintain the processes of life. These occur in our approximately thirty or so trillion human cells. What we should also appreciate is that a huge number of biochemical reactions are also occurring in our gut organisms. This does, of course, matter tremendously since, unlike our human cells, our gut organisms—our "second set of genes"—can be quickly changed. So indeed we are not totally determined by our birth genes.

It really doesn't matter much whether we prefer not to think about this. It's biology, and it's reality. We often think in terms of the cleaning product advertisements that imply all bacteria are bad. Of course, that's quite wrong. All bacteria are not bad, and many are extremely beneficial.

The right gut microorganisms are essential to our life and heart health.

Many antibiotics will markedly change the population of our gut bacteria, mostly for the worse, requiring reintroduction of good microorganisms. Sugary foods and carbohydrates that quickly turn to sugar favor the growth of unhealthy microorganisms in our gut, so we are well advised to limit our intake of such foods.

Probiotics

Probiotics is the term given to a collection of good bacteria.

Taking oral probiotics to help colonize our gut with beneficial microorganisms is helpful in our heart health.

Predominance of bad gut bacteria can result in may common symptoms including bloating, diarrhea, crampy pain, and constipation. There are some "diseases" that are named to account for the multiple symptoms that are partly produced by bad gut bacteria. Irritable bowel syndrome, colitis, spastic colitis, etc. etc.

The Human Microbiome Project

The Human Microbiome Project is an amazing recent scientific endeavor looking at gut organisms. We should all be aware of the truths of this effort. Our gut organisms are a critical component of our health. Some gut organisms are proving to be more heart-healthy than others. Lactobacilli Reuteri and Rhamnosus fall into this category. Unfortunately, there is no clear and easy way to measure this problem presently. The best we can do is to estimate how bad the symptoms are.

Beneficial microorganisms are called probiotics.

Common food sources of probiotics include:

- Sauerkraut

- Pickled vegetables

- Fermented cheeses

- Kefir—a fermented milk product that provides probiotics and beneficial yeast. Many of us like the tartness, good flavors including blueberry can cut it if desired

- Tempeh, miso, kimchi, and kombucha tea are good sources for those who choose Asian foods.

Capsules can provide an effective dose of active probiotic organisms. A reasonable estimate is that probiotic capsules should provide 30 to 50 billion colony forming units (CFUs.) Some probiotics require refrigeration after opening to decrease the degradation of the organisms. Blister packed capsules and other preparations can be at room temperature until used.

Prebiotics

Additionally, it's good to understand that good microbes prosper when they can access fiber. It's the scaffolding that lets them thrive. The term "prebiotic" is often used for this component of nutrition.

Non-Digestible Fibers Are Prebiotics

Natural fiber sources include:

- Onions

- Leeks

- Asparagus

- Bananas

Psyllium based products are a convenient way to ingest good fiber. Commercially available psyllium based products include Metamucil, Konsyl, and Benefiber.

In all cases, it is best to start with small amounts to avoid bloating. Soluble fiber has the additional quality of lowering LDL cholesterol.

Fortunately, part of the answer to beating heart disease is simple. Take in good fiber and beneficial organisms.

Taking both prebiotics and probiotics in an effective form will help achieve good nutrition, can decrease inflammation, and maintain healthy blood vessels.

Yes, we have the guts to fight heart disease.

~~~

DRILL DOWNS

Drill Down 1:

These microorganisms make up an average of 2% of our body mass. That's two pounds for a 100-pound person and four pounds for a 200-pound person.

~~~

In the next section we address one of the things we have always associated with heart trouble: Activity. What new information do we have about this? And what do we have to do to make it work for us?

~~~

References and Further Reading:

1. The Human Intestinal Microbiome in Health and Disease
Susan V. Lynch, Ph.D., and Oluf Pedersen, M.D., D.M.Sc.
N Engl J Med 2016; 375:2369-2379 December 15, 2016doi: 10.1056/Nejmra1600266

2. Campbell JH, O'Donoghue P, Campbell AG, Schwientek P, Sczyrba A, Woyke T, Söll D, Podar M. Uga is an additional glycine codon in uncultured sr1 bacteria from the human microbiota. Proc natl acad sci usa 2013, mar 18. Pmid: 23509275

3. https://www.NIH.Gov/news-events/news-releases/nih-human-microbiome-project-defines-normal-bacterial-makeup-body

4. Jones M, Martoni C, Prakash S. Cholesterol lowering and inhibition of sterol absorption by lactobacillus reuteri ncimb: a randomized controlled trial. Eur j clin nutr. 2012;66(11):1234-41

ACTIVITY

SITTING EQUALS SMOKING

WE CAN ACTIVELY FIGHT HEART DISEASE

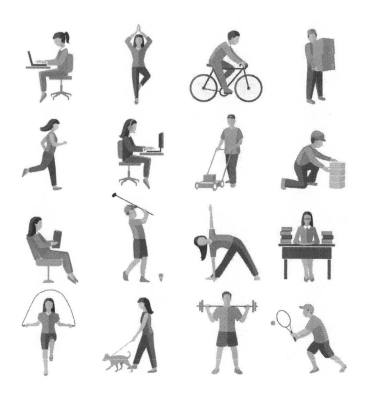

This is not even a subject up for debate. We must stay active or decline. We all know this, but what's new?

Have you ever heard that sitting is as bad as smoking? Yes, the effect is that important. The science is compelling, showing over 100% increased risk of bad heart-related events with an inactive day-to-day life.

We might blow up like a blob or dwindle to nothing, but inactivity is certainly the choice to decline. Inaction is just as much a choice as action is.

We must simply be active. Whatever we want to do is good. From walking to gardening, to sports, to standing instead of sitting, to walking in place, the important thing is to just do something.

Here again, the details get many of us off the path. We must simply find whatever works for us individually and is the most enjoyable, thus becoming sustainable. Whether our action is to stand rather than sit when talking on the phone (good) or to do HIT—high intensity interval training—(best), it's all about getting it done and choosing what is sustainable.

Attitude is everything when it comes to activity. It's not about the exercise bike you don't have, the gym membership you can't afford, or whatever barrier we allow our mind or inner critic to set up. There is no magic bullet here or elsewhere! We must simply develop the habits of being more active with what we have now.

This concept of the benefits of simply being active is being confirmed. For further research into this area look into the acronym "NEAT." It stands for non-exercise activity thermogenesis. (4)

~~~

In our next chapter, Heart Health Today reviews current data on nutrition. We've all seen "Heart Healthy" labels on many foods. The latest on that is next.

~~~

References and Further Reading:

Stamatakis E, et al. Screen-based entertainment time, all-cause mortality, and cardiovascular events: Population-based study with ongoing mortality and hospital events follow-up. Journal of the American College of Cardiology. 2011;57:292

Dunstan DW, et al. Television viewing time and mortality: The Australian Diabetes, Obesity and Lifestyle Study (AusDiab). Circulation. 2010;121:384

Li, I., Mackey, M., Foley, B., Pappas, E., Edwards, K., Chau, J., Engelen, L., Voukelatos, A., Whelan, A., Bauman, A., Stamatakis, E., et al (2017). Reducing Office Workers' Sitting Time at Work Using Sit-Stand Protocols: Results From a Pilot Randomized Controlled Trial. Journal of Occupational and Environmental Medicine, 59(6), 543-549, June 2017

Non-exercise activity thermogenesis (NEAT) Levine, James A., Best Practice & Research Clinical Endocrinology & Metabolism, 2002Dec; Volume 16, Issue 4, 679–702

Arnson Y, Rozanski A, Gransar H, et al. Impact of exercise on the relationship between CAC scores and all-cause mortality. J Am Coll Cardiol Img 2017;10:1461-8

NUTRITION

We Can Eat Our Way to Better Heart Health

This is one of the most complex and confusing parts of heart disease prevention. Theories and all manner of good and bad information abound. We endeavor to bring a current and focused perspective to all that's out there. We feel that clearly there are more than a few ways careful nutrition leads to heart health.

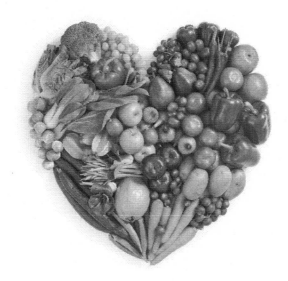

First Remember What We Are as Humans:

The building blocks composing us humans are the elements—predominately carbon, hydrogen, oxygen, and nitrogen. (1) After our human DNA arranges these elements in particular sequences and designs, we are the soup of hundreds of thousands of biochemical reactions that comprise our human biology.

Let's save the current information on what our skin absorbs and what we breathe in for another time. For the most part, the maxim is true:

"WE ARE WHAT WE EAT."

The old computer maxim is also true:

My wife, on her way out the door, just said, "I'll see what healthy things I can find for us." As she often does, she comes back with wonderful choices. From time to time, we enjoy going out to see what we can find as well.

Farm stands are a favorite with locally grown vegetables and fruits. The docks and markets where fresh seafood from uncontaminated waters can be found are a real find.

Supermarkets are a mixed bag. As we enter the store, we often first find the fresh produce our hearts love. A myriad of non-starchy, heart-healthy vegetables hits our eye. We are careful to choose fruits only in moderation. As we continue along the outside rim of the store, we find other choices which are more or less healthy, including fish, poultry, grass-fed meats, and butter as well as some other healthy spreads. Various types of milk (almond is a favorite), extra virgin olive oil, vinegars, nuts, and a few heart-healthy nutrition bars are often found in the adjacent aisles. We choose whole grain products only in moderation.

Simply put, fresh, whole foods are the best finds. If we have the inclination to be plant-based and meat and dairy-free, that can be a good choice.

For the most part, the central parts of the supermarkets are disaster areas, which are crammed with packaged goods and beverages. They manage to hide large amounts of the most unhealthy ingredients available. These include trans fats, high fructose corn syrup, and sugar and sugar equivalents. Conveniently packaged in brightly colored, attractive containers, they are difficult to avoid. The checkout line truly traps the youngest and most easily influenced of us with an absolute rash of sugar in one form or another.

Simply going to the healthiest areas first and making the good choices there often helps.

Contamination:

We must be vigilant that our foods are not contaminated with pesticides, antibiotics, or heavy metals. Selecting certain organically grown products can help avoid most pesticide and antibiotic ingestion.

Let's remember to avoid antibiotic and pesticide-contaminated foods.

The heavy metal mercury is found in certain fish, mainly the largest ones at the top of the food chain and those from contaminated waters. Lead is present in certain waters. There is actually also a small amount of arsenic in certain prepared foods. All these "heavy metals" impair some of our biological reactions and are correctly considered "poisonous" to humans.

The ideal level of all of these is zero. Blood tests are available to check out our heavy metal levels and may well be worth the price.

Let's remember the ideal level of mercury, lead, and arsenic in the human body is: **Zero.**

What Makes Fat:

"BREAD GOES TO SUGAR AND SUGAR GOES TO FAT!"

We were having lunch after golf when one of my buddies ordered a salad. He said he had stopped eating bread. When I asked why, he said, "bread goes to sugar and sugar goes to fat." He is very accomplished in his own field, which happens to be a unique field of flavor science, not specifically health. I was totally amazed by his insight. "You got it right!" I said. Ninety-nine percent of people would have said "fat goes to fat."

Let's remember, excess sugars, carbohydrates, and starches drive the production

of body fat more than the fat we eat does. ***(See Drill Down 1)***

It is perhaps natural to think that the fat we see and eat in meat and fish is primarily what is making us fat. The biology, however, is more complex than that.

We can forget the thousands of organic chemistry reactions that are involved. Eating the good fats and not the sugars or the carbs that quickly go to sugar is a road to better health, which equals less plaque in our arteries.

Getting down to the practicality of it, we all know most fast food sells well not because it is nutritious or healthy but precisely because it is fast and often cheap. It immediately answers two of our major concerns: time and money. The sad part is that the impulsive choice ends up being a short-term gain for a larger long-term loss of both time and money. Consider the cost of healthcare individually and as nations. There is absolutely no way we can afford it if the root causes of this disease are not conquered.

We Must Avoid Riding on the Sugar Roller Coaster

Sugary foods or foods that are quickly converted to sugar by our chemistry result in a rapid blood sugar spike. Insulin quickly reacts to push that sugar into cells and lowers blood sugar. However, in a couple of hours, the overshoot to a low blood sugar produces an intense craving and hunger. We quickly eat or drink some more to satisfy that uncomfortable feeling, and that is almost always some of the same stuff. The end result over a day is, of course, that we eat or drink large amounts of sugar, ending up with a daily ride on a sugar roller coaster. (See Drill Down 2)

One unique way we've noted that some of us deal with this uncomfortable feeling of being suddenly hungry is to have a giant soda on hand at all times, constantly sipping on it. We see this especially when stopping at a gas station/convenience store. They take selling sugar to a whole new level. The huge displays are almost all sugar in one form or another. Sweetened soda or "energy drinks" are choices that appear to work well in relieving the sugar-hunger cycle, as the constantly replaced blood sugar can never get too low. Frequently choosing this option can make us temporarily content and satisfied, however, it is also evident that we then wish we had less trouble fitting behind the wheel.

Healthier but certainly more difficult-to-find choices are a low-sugar snack bar, a bag of nuts, a glass of bottled water or unsweetened green tea.

The body needs sugar for our immediate energy needs, but quickly stores any excess in the form of—are you ready for this—the "F" word: Fat.

Starch

So what exactly is a "starch?" To paraphrase Wikipedia, a starch is "a carbohydrate consisting of a large number of glucose (sugar) units joined by (chemical) bonds." In other words, it is just a whole bunch of sugar put together!

Starch is most commonly found in staple foods such as potatoes, wheat, corn, and rice. Note here that grains are starches and to a large extent just a bunch of sugar. Those who prepare our livestock for market have learned long ago that feeding grain in abundance is the best way to add on pounds and profit.

Again, isn't it the fat we eat that results in our fat? Simply put, no, it's not. Mostly it's the excess sugars, carbohydrates, and starches consumed in the typical two-hour cycle that does it. Excess non-vegetable carbs and starches make us fat!

Sugary processed foods, flours, and starches such as potatoes, white rice, and corn, are inflammatory, addicting, and make us fat.
We should not take in more than our immediate energy need requires.

Obesity as a Disease

In our great effort as a society to organize and categorize, symptoms have been grouped into "diseases." Actually, the term "disease" is used so freely that at times it is totally confusing. Diseases have at times been created out of attempts to understand and categorize dysfunctional biochemistry, but primarily come from a need for philanthropic efforts, marketing medications, and administering medical payments. That's all good, but we should understand that the term often has very little, if anything, to do with the root cause of the disorder.

Most recently, obesity has been designated as a "disease." This categorization serves to allow medical payments for services related to managing health, and at least serves to focus on this condition. However, the guilt, stigma, and other societal crap that surrounds this symptom of "disease" need to be put aside. We need to focus on what causes obesity and use the knowledge to our advantage as we choose. As an aside, we certainly don't need to adversely judge others who are happy and accepting of this expression of their present biochemistry.

What we need to know is that excess carbohydrates get converted into body fat. Eating what we think of as fat is mostly not what makes us "fat." It is clearly—again a drumroll here—the excess of non-vegetable carbohydrates.

Knowing this simple truth clarifies our best nutritional choices.

Another useful thought:

It's what we eat first that matters.

Merely starting with the good foods satisfies our hunger!

"Sugar-Free" or "No Sugar Added"—Not Exactly!

Sugar Alcohols

"Sugar-free" chewing gum, soft drinks, ice creams, candies, and cookies often contain sugar alcohols.

Sugar alcohols appear on these and many other processed food labels as one of those many mysterious ingredients. These include mannitol, sorbitol, xylitol, lactitol, HSH (hydrogenated starch hydrolysates,) glycerol (glycerine or glycerin,) isomalt, maltitol, and erythritol.

They are employed because they have about half the sweetness of sugar. Sugar alcohols actually also have half of the calories. The chemical structure of sugar alcohols only resembles what is commonly classified as a true sugar, thus technically and somewhat deceptively allowing the name "sugar-free."

The name sugar alcohol might also lead to the idea that these ingredients contain ethanol, the type in alcoholic beverages. They do not.

Except for erythritol, sugar alcohols are not well absorbed in the small intestine and thus can lead to bloating, abdominal cramps and diarrhea. Some people note these products do not satisfy their hunger.

Sugar alcohols are found naturally, only to a small degree, in sweet potatoes, olives, asparagus, and carrots.

Sugar alcohols are not to be confused with artificial sweeteners. Aspartame, saccharin, sucralose, and acesulfame-k do not have calories, but certainly do have their own major health concerns associated with them. We choose to avoid these as well.

Let's remember sugar alcohols occur in many processed foods and have half of the calories of sugar

The Carb, Fat, Protein Confusion

A classic way of looking at our nutrition is to classify foods into carbs, fats, and proteins. This classification is way too broad to allow us to plan good heart-healthy nutrition. Biology demands we understand food in a slightly more specific way.

There are good fats and bad fats, good carbs and bad carbs, and the right amount of protein for optimal heart health.

Carbs:

Good carbs are non-starchy vegetables and high-fiber grains.

Bad carbs are starchy and those that are stripped of nutrients. (So-called "refined carbs" is one of the greatest misnomers of our time. Depleted carbs would be a better name.)

Some of us may recall the lyrics to Billy Joel's big hit "Uptown Girl." As a downtown guy, he references her high class "white bread world." In the last century, we were sold on the white color of grain products being the cleaner, better choice. That was certainly sad and fortunately, most of that outdated perception has changed. The lectin story may change it even further. We will be following up on this at hearthealthtoday.com.

Fats:

Good fats are omega-3 fats and a few omega-6 and 9 fats.

Bad fats are those leading to inflammation in the body, including all trans fats. Most vegetable oils promote the inflammation we should seek to avoid. Some do this more than others.

Proteins:

Proteins are essential components of our being. Getting the variety and proper amount is the important thing.

Cholesterol in the Diet.

Twentieth-century humorist Will Rogers said it best.

> *"It ain't what you don't know that gets you into trouble. It's what you know for sure that just ain't so."*

For years we knew for sure that it was the cholesterol we ate that gave us heart disease. However, in 2015 even the previously, sluggishly responsive U.S. Government Dietary Guidelines Advisory Committee removed the decades-long recommendation for restricting cholesterol intake. Continuing scientific studies put an end to an era! We should embrace the science of our new century. (3)

We will spare the reader the somewhat dull scientific papers showing this is true.

Those seeking a few very readable references in this regard should consider reading Nina Teicholz, "The Big Fat Surprise", Mark Hyman, "Good Fat, Bad Fat" and the following link: https://healthimpactnews.com/2014/time-magazine-we-were-wrong-about-saturated-fats/

It's clear we need to eat certain essential fats for our biochemical system to function optimally. Eaten in reasonable portions, they will not make us "fat." We must always remember that it's the excess of low-fiber carbohydrates that will result in excess "fat."

Most people think of fat as animal fat in meat. Biologically, however, we should think of this as a larger category, including plant as well as animal fat. The key, however, is to maintain an optimal balance of good fats.

Blood Work for Today

Lipid science is very complex, so consider having a detailed lipid test. Low LDL particle number is one current indicator for good heart health. Like LDL, HDL is a large category and the characteristics of various subsets are now coming to light. Overall, high HDL has been considered good, but high HDL particle number may well be a better indicator of the desirable level than total HDL. The smallest HDL fraction is likely beneficial as it is the initial particle in removing cholesterol. As a detailed drill down, we would recommend studying the work of Dr. Thomas Dayspring who has a knack for clarifying a very complex segment of our biology. (10)

The Low-Fat Label Trap

What about all that stuff we've been told over the past several years that low fat is good and eating fat is bad? It sort of implies that eating low-fat food will make us less fat. Let's just make a long history lesson very short: a generalized fear of eating fat and cholesterol is very misguided. Our information is now much more detailed and researched than what was reflected in the outdated recommendations of the '90s.

The many foods that are marketed as "low fat" are a trap with regard to preventing heart disease. Certainly, the products are low in fat, but this is largely accomplished by replacing the fat with sugar. Ironically, the sugar actually makes us fat. This substitution does more harm than good for our heart health.

Let's also remember that replacing total fat or saturated fat with carbohydrates is not associated with reduced risk of heart and blood vessel disease.

It is worth repeating that many processed foods labeled as "low fat" have had the fat replaced with sugar. This substitution makes us fat and does more harm than good for our heart health. (See Drill Down 3)

Good Food and Bad Food:

Again, one way to understand food is to categorize it into protein, carbohydrate, or fat. Beyond that, presumptions, incorrect conclusions, imaginative marketing, misconceptions, and general confusion reign.

The area of fats in the diet is getting a new look. The old ways of evaluating this were based mostly on how easy it was to do the blood test like cholesterol. Thus total cholesterol put many bad and good fats in the same bin. Measuring on the basis of density, high (HDL) and low (LDL) is easy to do and much data was accumulated. That helped to some degree but still lumped some harmful and beneficial molecules together.

Looking at this complex question, one of the clearest ways to unravel it may well be to simply look at good and bad fats.

Good Fats and Bad Fats:

We now know that the enemies are bad fat (all trans fat and some other fats)

The good fats are mostly omega 3 fats. This biological fact is so important, we choose to go into it in further detail with our I CAN DO acronym. We never cease to be amazed at this part of our biochemistry and how understanding it can improve our heart health.

Good Carbs and Bad Carbs:

Let's remember, high-fiber carbs are good and refined, sugary carbs are bad.

Good carbs are high-fiber carbs

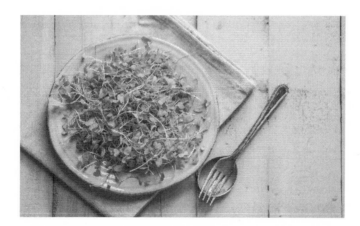

Good Protein and Bad Protein:

We suspect animal products used in moderation can be a healthy choice.

Good protein is uncontaminated vegetable and seafood protein. Some may choose animal protein in moderation.

If we wish to undertake the rigors of maintaining a vegan diet, there is evidence that it can provide an additional level of protection from inflammation for some of us. (6) Our biology also clearly tells us that supplementation with certain nutrients makes sense with this choice. B12 and algal EPA & DHA are included here.

Many of us are overfed and undernourished.

So What Do We Eat?

Low net carbs, high good fat nutrition is an excellent choice

It limits the sugar spikes in blood that are so harmful to us.

Fiber carbs are "good carbs" and don't count in totaling any carb limits. They are not quickly digested and therefore don't rapidly add to the blood sugar spike. These can include many nutritious vegetables and fruits.

Low net carbs (fiber carbs don't count), high good fat nutrition is an excellent choice. We should eat enough carbohydrate/starch only for our immediate energy needs. Include nutritious vegetables of all types, as much as we want.

Good proteins need to be included.

Fish-wild caught salmon and mackerel are best.

Meat and dairy protein in moderation can be a good choice and grass fed is best. Those who are allergic to dairy or cannot properly digest dairy should consider almond milk and olive oil based spreads.

The best portion size may well be one that fits in our hand.

Good fats can take the form of nuts, especially walnuts, almonds, and pecans, (not peanuts), sunflower seeds, extra virgin olive oil, wild caught salmon, and mackerel. Avocados are also a very satisfying source of good fat and are an amazing hunger-killer.

Trying to change a diet that is deeply ingrained into an individual by culture, habit, and example can be very challenging but well worth it. The irony of the term "ingrained" should not be lost on us.

Consider that all of us are descended from hunter-gatherers who spent most of their time getting food. Today, it is very important that we devote enough time and effort in getting the most heart-healthy food we can find.

All Those Many Diets

We believe a few of the so-called "diets" currently popularized have a lot of merit. Among them are the totally whole food, plant-based diet, the Dash diet, the South Beach

Diet, and the best-studied one, the Mediterranean Diet. We believe there is not one, but several ways to get heart-healthy nutrition.

What is also clear is that nutrition science still has much to elucidate about what we call food. While we do have some answers and general ways to proceed, we should not be so arrogant as to say we have all the answers here. The roles of soy and lectins, in particular, are certainly still under investigation.

The Mediterranean way is a heart healthy choice for us.

The Mediterranean Diet now has abundant evidence as being very heart healthy. It is based on extra virgin olive oil, fresh fruits, legumes, nuts, and some whole grains. It includes many vegetables other than corn, rice, or potatoes. Moderate fish, poultry, seafood, cheese, and yogurt are part of this approach. Also advised are lower intakes of red meat and eggs. Herbs are a good substitute for salt. Luckily for us, incorporating even one or two of the components of the diet into a daily routine can have a beneficial effect.(8)

Relatively new to the market are microgreens: collections of very nutrient-rich plants 1 to 3 inches tall. These are an excellent choice for inclusion in any nutrition program. (11)

Some of Our Thoughts on an Easy, Middle of the Road Approach:

WHAT TO BUY	WHAT NOT TO BUY
Uncontaminated food	Contaminated food (toxin containing)
Foods improving our biochemistry	Foods impairing our biochemistry

CARBS:

Colored vegetables	Sugar in all its forms
Broccoli, cauliflower	Bread
Onions, radishes	Potatoes

Mushrooms	Flour based groceries
Fresh fruit in moderation, whatever is appealing	Corn
Microgreens	Cakes
	Cookies
	Pastries

FATS:

Grass fed beef	Greasy food
Wild caught fish high in omega-3	Some saturated fats
Olive oil or anything prepared with it	
Avocado	
Omega 3 eggs	
Butter, preferably grass-fed	

PROTEINS:

Poultry prepared with lemon, olive oil	High-fat meats
Tomatoes, or any colored vegetable. Poultry not fed with lectin or soy is likely better.	

Fish, preferable high in omega-3

Lean pork and grass-fed beef

Vegetable protein

High-quality protein shakes (low sugar content)

A good food shake mix is often a superb choice

Spices for flavor are healthy, especially oregano, cilantro, and turmeric

Micronutrient supplements (these can quickly and efficiently provide us with

many of the building blocks we need
for better heart health)

BEVERAGES:

Regular coffee (not more than 4 cups
per day)

Green tea

Filtered water

Pomegranate juice

Almond milk

Electrolyte drinks when training

Sugar drinks

"Diet" drinks

Sugar added juices

Sodas

What to Order:

We heard a very effective phrase when a friend was giving their dinner order. "No starch,
please. I'd like double vegetables or fruit." Their simple request was easily
accommodated.

This is a suggestion that when employed will lead to better heart health…no guarantees
you will be seen as skinny.

~~~

DRILL DOWNS

Drill Down 1:

The process is known as lipogenesis. Wikipedia defines this for us:

"Lipogenesis is the process by which acetyl-coa is converted to fatty acids. The former is
an intermediate stage in metabolism of simple sugars, such as glucose, a source of
energy of living organisms. Through lipogenesis and subsequent triglyceride
synthesis, the energy can be efficiently stored in the form of fats."

Drill Down 2:

The "sugar roller coaster" story has to do with our hormones and how several of them work to signal hunger or the opposite of hunger, which is "feeling full" or satiety. Check out ghrelin, leptin, and insulin among others (9)

Drill Down 3:

meats   *beans, legumes?*

Evidence has also shown that replacing saturated fats with carbohydrates reduces blood levels of total and LDL-cholesterol, but increases blood levels of triglycerides and reduces high-density lipoprotein-cholesterol (HDL-cholesterol). Replacing total fat or saturated fats with carbohydrates is not associated with reduced risk of heart and blood vessel disease. (15)

~~~

In the next section, we will boil all this down to the basics and use the KISS principle attributed to the U.S. Navy in the '60s (Keep It Simple Stupid).

~~~

References and Further Reading:

1. Bruna Fernandes Azevedo, Lorena Barros Furieri, Franck Maciel Peçanha, et al., "Toxic Effects of Mercury on the Cardiovascular and Central Nervous Systems," Journal of Biomedicine and Biotechnology, vol. 2012, Article ID 949048, 11 pages, 2012. Doi: 10.1155/2012/949048

2. AHA SCIENTIFIC STATEMENT
https://doi.org/10.1161/01.CIR.0000019552.77778.04
Circulation. 2002;106:523-527 Originally published July 23, 2002

3. U.S. Department of Health and Human Services and U.S. Department of Agriculture. *2015–2020 Dietary Guidelines for Americans*. 8th Edition. December 2015. Available at https://health.gov/dietaryguidelines/2015/guidelines/

4. Sugar and Cardiovascular Disease
A Statement for Healthcare Professionals From the Committee on Nutrition of the Council on Nutrition, Physical Activity, and Metabolism of the American Heart Association
Barbara V. Howard, Judith Wylie-Rosett
https://doi.org/10.1161/01.CIR.0000019552.77778.04
Circulation. 2002;106:523-527

5. http://www.foodinsight.org/articles/sugar-alcohols-fact-sheet

6. The effect of a vegan versus AHA Diet in coronary artery disease (EVADE CAD) trial: Study design and rationale
Shah, B; Ganguzza, L; Slater, J; Newman, J D; Allen, N; Fisher, E; Larigakis, J; Ujueta, F; Gianos, E; Guo, Y; Woolf, K
Contemporary clinical trials communications. 2017 December. 8 (pp): 90-98

7. http://dx.doi.org/10.1016/j.atherosclerosis.2011.04.026

8. http://www.atherosclerosis-journal.com/article/S0021-9150(11)00372-8/fulltext

9. Journal of Pedi Austin and Marks. Hormonal Regulators of Appetite Endocrinology; 2008,2009 141753

10. Dayspring, T Understanding HDL Complexities
www.lipidcenter.com/pdf/Understanding_HDL_Complexities.pdf

11. Xiao,Z; Lester,G.; Luo,Y.; Wang,Q. Assessment of Vitamin and Carotenoid Concentrations of Emerging Food Products: Edible Microgreens. Journal of Agricultural and Food Chemistry 2012,60,7644-7651

12. Hung, H. C.; Joshipura, K. J.; Jiang, R.; Hu, F. B.; Hunter, D.; Smith-Warner, S. A.; Colditz, G. A.; Rosner, B.; Spiegelman, D.; Willett, W. C. Fruit and vegetable intake and risk of major chronic disease. J. Natl. Cancer Inst. 2004, 96, 1577-1584

13. Craig, W.; Beck, L. Phytochemicals: health protective effects. Can
J. Diet Pract. Res. 1999, 60, 78-84

14. Rice-Evans, C.; Miller, N. J. Antioxidants - the case for fruit and vegetables in the diet. Br. Food J. 1995, 97, 35-40

15. U.S. Department of Health and Human Services and U.S. Department of Agriculture. *2015–2020 Dietary Guidelines for Americans.* 8th Edition. December 2015. Available at https://health.gov/dietaryguidelines/2015/guidelines/

NOW LET'S GET TO IT

We have emphasized what we feel are 6 of the most important factors to build heart health.

I Reduce harmful Inflammation—do it with anti-inflammatory nutrition and consider supplements to reach and maintain our hsCRP goal.

C Control gut health. Attain and maintain healthy gut organisms with nutrition, prebiotics, probiotics from food, and, if desired, supplement sources.

A ACTIVITY is a key component. We understand now that this is ANY type of activity. Walk in place, take the stairs, take a walk, ride a bike etc, etc. They ALL work. We know success depends on monitoring progress and results.

N NUTRITION. We know that nutrition is a big part of the answer. This is an ongoing quest to find better and better programs with the variety that can be accepted by any one of us. We have referenced the programs we feel are on the right track and some of the best individual food choices. More on this important topic is to be found on our website and further publications.

D An excellent vitamin D3 level is a cornerstone of good heart health. It's simple enough and just as critical as it is simple.

O Omega-3s have been proven to be vital to heart health. We employ them with our nutrition and supplementation to achieve our goals.

Let's remember the DO part is critical.

New information is constantly becoming available at an ever-increasing speed. We will continue to update our perspective on all of this on our website:

HEARTHEALTHTODAY.COM

Cultivate willpower, that massive, creative force that the creator built into you.

Do not let it remain flabby, but strengthen it by use and exercise.

~Norman Vincent Peale

DISCLAIMER 2

The information provided herein is for informational purposes only. This information is shared as a product of the authors' personal quest for heart health and our personal perspective. The authors expressly disclaim responsibility for any adverse events resulting from use of any of the information provided. Each of us is alone responsible for our own decisions. The reader assumes the risk of any benefit or injury. No health benefits are guaranteed. If you do not accept this view, please do not avail yourself of any of this information.

Implementation of any information provided into any personal regimen must be done only in consultation with, and clearance by, your physician or health care professional. You must not rely on any information from this publication or website as an alternative to advice from your healthcare professional. If you have, or suspect you have, a medical problem, promptly contact your healthcare provider immediately and proceed under their guidance.

The information provided DOES NOT create a doctor-patient relationship between you and any of the health care professionals involved.

Any information or statement regarding any dietary supplements are not intended to diagnose, cure, prevent, or treat any disease and have not been evaluated by the Food and Drug Administration. References to particular products are for adults only. Children, pregnant women, and nursing mothers must in particular follow the specific advice of their health care provider. All product labels must be carefully reviewed for safety information, dose, administration, and contraindications. HEART HEALTH TODAY, LLC may benefit from the sales of these products or services.

Our mission is to bring the reader our perspective on today's scientific information concerning heart health. The authors have learned, and to continue to learn, from a multitude of conferences, lectures, personal discussions, and reviews of the literature. No independent verification of any of the data herein has been performed. History has taught us well that the field of health is constantly changing and being updated with new information and research that may either confirm or refute previous conclusions. We expressly disclaim any errors in the literature. This work is the authors' personal understanding and interpretation. The readers should verify all information through their own personal research.

ABOUT THE AUTHOR

Don Zone has been pursuing the truths of human biology since childhood. His professional training with a B.S. in preprofessional studies and M.D. have allowed him contact with a multitude of those pursuing similar interests and they are in some degree authors of this work. A career in the subspecialty of cardiology has provided the opportunity to be involved with those suffering the ravages of heart disease. The current emphasis of his team has been guided by the appreciation of how absolutely necessary it is to understand the root causes of heart disease in order to prevent and reverse this villain.

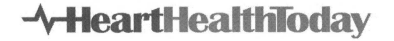

Made in the USA
Columbia, SC
06 April 2019